KICKITWELLorELSE

KICKITWELLorelse

Be Healthy and Attractive
Quit Smoking

ARNOUX PRINCE

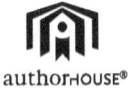

authorHOUSE®

AuthorHouse™
1663 Liberty Drive
Bloomington, IN 47403
www.authorhouse.com
Phone: 1-800-839-8640

Published by AuthorHouse 2/6/2013

ISBN: 978-1-4817-0401-4 (sc)
ISBN: 978-1-4817-0402-1 (e)

Table of Contents

Forewords

Human beings have been put through unnecessary struggle. I hope everybody would get off this kind of bandwagon some day.

The writer of kickitwellorelse is referring to 'the struggle to survive propagated by some of the proponents of the theory of the jungle or "survived the fittest"It implies that only big and strong animals survive. It implies that some wars are justified on the ground that the dead ones were not strong enough to survive, on the ground that war is natural thing to do. The theory doesn't make sense, obviously. It doesn't reflect any kind of reality, never have, and never will. For from the beginning of creation there were small weak and big and strong animals on the earth. Small(or weak) animals still exist now. No, the big ones haven't eaten them, for one thing. Small and weak animals and big and strong animals were created to survive. They do.

We, human beings, were all born with a psyche in which there are the will, the creative mind, etc., to guide us, help us find the solutions of problems that we face, although the ego, an excessive materialism prevent us from using this extraordinary tool.

It is true that war and famine are still with us, sign of human struggle. But that is rather the result of alienation, personal disharmony. They are nothing natural as the theory would like you to believe. They are not supposed to be as the theory implies. Evolutionism deriving from creationism fathers the theory "survived the fittest ". Those two predominant doctrines are harmful to us most of the time. They create in us conflicts and contradictions.Someone says: "War is individual conflict magnified in a million" .

No wonder you want to give up a habit and don't succeed under the spell of these doctrines.

You have learned to smoke in a society where it was cool (even now too, a little bit) to display such behavior, in one hand. In the other the same society is saying that it is not something to do by banishing it in public places.

The author of kickitwellorelse himself was in the same kind of situation once. One day I woke up and quit.

Instead of trying to be happy, we see strange things happening to us on this planet of ours. Buildings have been blown up without any consideration for life. Civilian human beings, having nothing to do with army, just trying to live their lives, in a supermarket, in a bus going home. Bang! they are dead or wounded. Isn't that sad and repulsive at the same time ? There is no bravery there. If you want to be brave you alone would attack an army.

On the other hand, if you know a place is deadly contentious, you still go and settle there, you are looking for trouble .You are saying that violence is the way ro settle differences.

In one hand, you are trying to settle in their land, in the other you are destroying their buildings. They are already poor. Your behavior is bizarre and bound to create more violence.

Who knows what the real cause of something like September 11 could be? Most of the time it points rather to craziness, the absurd. Nonetheless, going to cellular level to explain events is something I tend to do once in a while. September 11 reminds me of journalist of everywhere, including Americans and Orientals. I hear and read in the news often that doing something extraordinary, like winning a jackpot, is equivalent to having an accident. But human beings do win jackpot everyday in the world. There is no research that links these winners with accident Journalists think like that because they are like the rest of us, they like to work, they like to have accident to report.

This desire is at cellular level, of course.

It is possible to think that September 11 as well as other big terrible events like that are caused by a desire of accident in human beings. Instead of accident, we should propagate that people are have extraordinary ability all the time, especially when they do something extraordinary like flying to the moon, winning first prizes.

Human beings are dying before their time is up, hook-up on habits that we can easily get rid of. Journalists, ex- premiers, ordinary men and women are dying because they are addicted to something which doesn't promote life in any way, which is not indipensable to life.

Many of us notice, at Christmas time, almost all of us are much happier. One of the girlfriends I had used to start buying Christmas gifts right from the beginning of spring. From that moment she was in the Christmas mood till the end of the year. She is probably not the only one who tries to prolong the Christmas party all through the year. That's the spirit we should all have; we should all try to be happy all try very often, as long as we keep in mind that life is dynamic, that nothing can be continuous We should all try to be happy a life time, all through the year not just at Christmas time. Some human beings try to be happy all the time, but the way they do it is questionable . How happy can we be after inhaling cigarette smoke?. Instead, we know it kills. Instead, two Chinese guys made a bet to see who, among the two was going to finish first smoking a pack a cigarettes. The winner fell to his death on the spot after finishing inhaling his pack of cigarettes.

After a few unsuccessful trials in my first attempts to quit smoking, I woke up one day and decided to give it up, to kick the habit away once and for all.

Afterwards, I thought researching the subject a little bit more and helping 'earthian' fellows in their own attempts to give up the mortifying habit.

That was in 1989. Teaching and other life involvements, feet sickness, death in the family prevented me from doing so before now

My other interests are writting books, creating an earthquacke detector, a machine capable of preventing big accident, another one capable of cahing criminal of big crimes on the spot,etc. It is not clear i'll be able to do any of it, having to focus still on matters of lesser importance.

I feel bad not having been able, to concentrate, to keep my attention on the big projects above when tere is an earthquacke, a big accident

Still most of the time, I am in a uplifting state of mind, for I have a lot to be grateful for, above all, being accepted as citizen of this big country such as Canada. By the way, I adore Ontarians(Although there is reason, also, to adore the inhabitants of the rest of Canada, the world) for the political soundness they applied when it was extremely needed and so keeping Canada together, from breaking into pieces. I feel I have to make this statement, because some of my westerners friends always poking fun at Ontarians.

Watching a TV report 23-04-2001 on a football player legend Terry Evanson and his family was another eye opener. According to it, in the middle of his extraordinary career, he has been involved in an accident. He recovered physically from it, but couldn't remember a damned thing from his past life, a kind of amnesia, and his entire mind was not functioning properly. Still no physical damage has been noticed in his brain after examination and tests. The diagnostic was that a sort of" diffused brain damaged" have caused his problem. According to the author of kickitwell, that diagnosis was like nothing, saying nothing, despite the good will and heart of the doctor who made it. Morsby's Medical Nursing and Allied Health Dictionary defines amnesia as being a lost of memory caused by brained damaged or a severe emotional trauma; Random Unabridged dictionary says; lost of large blocks of interrelated memories caused by brain injuries or shocks, etc. According to both dictionaries amnesia is caused also by mental factors alone. When there isn't brain damaged, why bringing brain in this sickness causation equation? The football player and his family were just very, very traumatized by the accident and the wrong it was going to inflict to them in terms of money, fame and health, . They were unable to face life in the new adverse conditions in which it placed them. The player and his family preferred to forget it all and took refuge in amnesia. In this case it was rather a "mind damaged". They were forced to see themselves no longer as an adorable football player family, but as a handicapped one, all of a sudden. They found it difficult to accept. After all post traumatic disorder is a very well known phenomenon.

Memory is related to brain like water is to electricity, but they are of different nature. It can be blocked, but not destroyed as the diagnostic implied, the mind being non-substantial and memory being part of the mind, memory is also non-substantial So memory blocks are not always linked to the brain as blackouts are not always s related to water that turns the turbine to make electricity. It may just be the result of a broken line.

I am not inventing the non-substantial nature of the mind and memory and all the other mind components. Humans have known this fact since first century, if not even a lot earlier than that, if not right from the start of human life. That's why we have the story of Santa bringing gifts to children in houses through the chimney. The non-substantial nature of Santa allows him to enter into the house through the chimney . In that sense, we should not only encourage children to believe the apparent mystery, but adults too.

Instead, belief in saying such as" What you see is what you get" ,"Seeing is believing" is what we encourage in people and what undermines health agents' vision, preventing them from seeing the clear picture of diseases and causes, when the latter are of concern at all in medicine? .No wonder the health system fails to help people like Terry Evanson.They are looking in the wrong direction. "Diffused brain damaged" sounds like a diagnostic made during the Stone Age by someone completely out of himself.

It was a moving experience to listen and watch this report not only for the suffering these families have endured, but also for the lamentable state in which medicine is still, compare to what it could be. They seem unable to distinguish the brain from the mind (Brain=animal organ, substantial, physical / Mind=part of people, part of the psyche, non-substantial, non-physical) and do better medicine. That reminds me of the news of research finding the spot in the where memory resides. How can it be there? It is not a substance, it's the mind. That makes me mad each time I hear it or read about it.

Mind you, misdiagnoses (are they debilitating need to create sickness at cellular level?) happen in psychiatry too. People spend a lot of times in psychiatric hospital for nothing or just because they are in the midst of psychic growth crisis. All in all big money is wasted on those misdiagnose.

Someone one's self is medicine at its best meaning that the higher you raise your consciousness the healthier you are. People heal themselves from cancer and other terminal sicknesses simply by envisioning a dream body in perfect health every day. They don't have to accept any imperfect diagnostic that is presented to them sometimes. Someone with self-knowledge and self-identification will have a healthy and rich attitude toward life, will use all his/her psychological processes and his body to keep her /himself healthy and rich as much as possible. You need to take your health matters in your own hands. We've just said more or less that each person is a better doctor to himself than the rest of all doctors in the whole world.Health is too private to leave it in the hand of big, almost abstract organization. Keep yourself away from hospital, institutionalized medicine as much as possible, traditional as well as alternative medicine. You see, medicinal practice is initiated to heal sick people. On the long run it becomes part of the sickness. For it is there to treat sick people. At cellular level, all hospital employees, everybody working in the health system want you to be sick. Otherwise, no job.

That said, it necessary for me to make a few brief comments taking into account that an introduction of a method to get rid of addiction is not a forum for any kind of philosophy. The first comment is in regard to doctors bashing because of possible intellectual jalousie noticeable in certain intellectual and political milieu (Recently Mr. Ralph Klein said on TV that "the doctors are in it for the money"). The problem mentioned above is not doctors bashing. Physicians and specialists in the medical field are like the rest of us somehow, some of them are fine persons(It's like the physician I see worries more about my health than myself), some less fine persons, some marginal or hooligans(like in the general population of any race there are about 80% of "good" people and between 1 to 20 % hooligans) . Hospital employees are not responsible for our sicknesses. Each person is responsible for himself, his own health or whatever. The kind of interest in sickness at cellular level awarded to all medical employees above is rather an existential one, unavoidable.

Neither is encouraging distance from institutionalized medicine a masculine, sexist motivation of the type: "It is a woman who goes to see a doctor" as it exist in society in general. The real motivation is the presence of the healer in everybody. I am asking myself: Why not suggesting to you to bring it to life, to exploit it?

Another comment is related to medical errors(medical errors or desire to create sickness at cellular level going bad?). This person publishes a book called: Medical Nightmares in which she stated that" 10 000 Canadians die of medical errors each year". I can remember watching a report on TV in 2000 on medical errors in England. In that report the number of deaths from medical errors were of course quite bigger, English population being bigger than Canadian's.

Another comment: Among these doctors who made these medical errors resulting in death aren't some doctor Kervokian's partisan?

Another comment: In doctors formation more psychology(Although the same problem exists in psychological practice too, to a lesser extent) is needed in other to prevent the formation of cellular nonsense in the health agent .Like it's said above, to function well someone has to be as close to himself as possible. Functioning like machines, we are in for non-sense.

Then, there is also that when accademic discipline and parapsychology unit in a person, he or she becomes almost like God.I know some.

Last comment: As an individual, I take the risk to appear insensitive by discouraging the use of the medical system in order to discard the latent intention to be sick. But any government which adopts such idea and tries to implement it "rush rush", a la va vite, without a very elaborate plan applied in a very slow fashion with previous education, would be judged likewise, insensitive, impeached, thrown out, erased from the political landscape in a very short while.

If the grant was awarded to you by the ministery, they would be able to read the above paragraph, instead of the bits of informations they've gathered from the letter asking for the grant which they applied in their health program anyway. Later the last thing I've heard, the ministry and the whole govenment was in serious trouble. Who has the last laugh?

I have the impression sometimes they don't want to help in the government, in order to be able to steal your ideas.

Another bugger is the so called reserahers of health who publish anything that comes to their mind with no link at all with research. Like the ones who plusfed that women who eat lot of vegetables won't have alzemeimer, women who eat spinach will have their memory improved. I get stomach cramp each time I hear one of those.

Alzemeimer is one of the so called functional diseases in psychology, and what I called socialization(that what the researches above do they confuse the rest of us) diseases. They are caused by confusion on the nature and the functions of the mind and the brain.

Part 1

The Issues

Chapter I

A) WHY ARE THERE UNSUCCESSFUL TRIALS TO QUIT SMOKING

The inventor of kickitwellorelse knows some of his friends (one friend is married, has permanent teaching job. He said "That the only pleasure I got" You thought "Wow!") are having trouble with their desire to quit smoking. You probably know more than one person successful in life but unsuccessful in their attempts to give up the habit. Million of people are unable to quit smoking on their own. Why is that? There is no definite answer to the question, but looking at how the habit is acquired will help find some of them.

How Is The Habit Acquired?

The writer of kickitwell started smoking when he was about 15 years old. His father and one of his elder brothers smoked cigar, cigarettes, tobacco in pipe, and raw tobacco. In Haiti they had the habit of not lighting their own cigarette or whatever they want to smoke. He doesn't know why but most of the time they asked someone else to do it for them, and that someone else happened to be younger ones such as myself and other brothers and sisters. He remembers to use a spoon to carry live coals from one point to the other. Cooking was done in a small house or in the yard separate from main house. After a number of times, I myself became a smoker.

According to Arthur H Cain, who wrote on he subject, people begin to smoke for various reasons of their own: It makes them feel grown up, cigarette can be stimulating, comforting, and pleasurable. Finally He says 'There has never been great taboos against smoking such as those against drinking and taking narcotics"'. Some religious groups object in principle to cigarette smoking and this is a valid consideration for the young members of those groups who are faced with the problem of whether or not to start smoking. 'But, by and large, the greatest of our population does not on moral grounds, frown on the use of cigarette, even by young persons in their teens'.

In Comprehensive Textbook of Psychiatry, by H.I. Kaplan, he writes that'The initiation seems to occur through social reinforcements. Almost nine out of ten teenagers who smoke tobacco report that at least one their best friends is a regular smoker. Non-smokers have exactly the opposite pattern'.

The passage about the social taboo above stirs in me several thoughts. Isn't it bizarre that society frowns on the use of cigarette but on alcohol, even though it's becoming more and more evident that alcohol is as harmful to our health than tobacco smoke? It is a temptation to try this explanation: tobacco smoking cannot divert anyone from his her social duties-work, family-while alcohol can. There is also the fact that alcohol is sold by the state in some countries, which is not the same for tobacco product. In these countries the habit of drinking is less discouraged, if not to say more encouraged, than the habit of smoking. But one can reason, consciously or at cellular level, that if the state is encouraging drinking which can destroyed the liver, cause deadly accidents, then it's ok to smoke, the dangerous effects of smoking being lot less apparent, might not even exist, according to a naive smoker pattern of thoughts. So some states in some countries also encourage smoking indirectly or not. So the mind being what it is, at cellular level you are invaded by suggestions to smoke, one reason why it is not easy for some people to give it up on their own.

These thoughts bring us back to the issue that is to say how do we acquire the habit of smoking? He would like to point out that smoking, at the end of it all, is a deliberate act. We are not born with some mysterious gene craving tobacco smoke.Mr.Cain wrote" No one ever developed a need or a craving for cigarettes unless he willfully get himself into the habit of smoking. Thi s, of course, does not necessarily prove that smoking is morally bad in itself, he knew some priests who are smokers. It is only merely pointed out here that the habit is an acquired one, does not constitute a bona fide need of the human organism.

According to Sydney Petrie in How to Quit Smoking in 3 Days,' the problem of smoking had become of such national concern that during the current year (1953) the United State Government as well as State Governments have allocated tens of millions of dollars for research that includes attention to the very serious problem of what methodologies are most effective in helping his citizens overcome this deadly habit, addiction, or call it what you will. 'Smoking "he continues, "has been recognized for the very serious problem that it is, not only by the thousands of investigators, from the medical, and psychological professional, but also the man/woman in the street".

According to what have been written above, the habit is acquired basically by social reinforcement and for various reasons of their own human beings have.

The author of Kickitwell thinks that a big part of the problem resides in that most of us is unfamiliar with very important facts and factors of life endangerment and the habit. Let's move on to the next chapter to find out.

Chapter II

B) HOW SMOKING ENDANGERS LIFE AND CONSEQUENCES OF SMOKING?

How Smoking Endangers Life?

To understand the effect of smoking in smokers 'lives, perhaps it necessary to know a little bit about the chemical elements there are in tobacco smoke. It is composed of many sorts of gases, some of which are very, very harmful to your health. That is the case of, for example, hydro cyanic acid, nitric oxide, nitrogen dioxide, acetone and ammonia. Among them, also, figures the colorless, odorless lethal carbon monoxide, on which science has zeroed in during the past few years and which makes up about 4% of cigarette smoke. According to Dr.Wilbert S. Aranov of the University of California **'This gas has been identified as contributing to heart attack and sudden coronary death in smokers'**. Furthermore, the US Surgeon General calculated **carbon monoxide is causing 170000 extra or premature heart attack deaths per year.**

Cigarette smoke is also composed of tar. A pack- a- day smoker inhales each year up to eight ounces, a full cup of tar in cigarette smoke. **Tar is a more cancer- causing agent than its parts, such as benzopyrene. Chronic** bronchitis and its steady companion, **emphysema--**, of which the US Surgeon General says cigarettes are the most important cause--**kill more than 30000 people and cause the lost of more than 35**

millions man-days of work per year. A little bit out dated for in Canada of only 30 millions plus people, around 1995 it was reported in the papers that 500000 people were dying each year from tobacco smoke. But tar can be found in products other than tobacco.

Also, in tobacco smoke there is nicotine, a very important part of the problem with smoking in general, for according to most smoking researchers, nicotine is responsible for addiction (the principle on the basis of which nicotine patch, nicoderm and some other quit smoking devices have been created, he thinks). From one to three milligrams of nicotine are in the average cigarette. As stimulant, the main effect of the nicotine is on the heart, the blood vessels, the digestive tracks and the kidneys. Nicotine raises the smoker's blood pressure and speeds up his pulse. It stimulates the flow of saliva and the general action of the lower digestive system. After that these bodily functions are depressed.

It stimulates the flow of saliva. Imagine being unable to stop one's flow of saliva and have to go hospital for that!!!.

Further more, there is an eye disease called tobacco ambylopia, caused by smoking which results in partial loss of sight without obvious damage to the retina or optical nerves. Some other diseases caused by smoking in literature are: lung cancer, heart palpitation, bladder cancer, intestinal mal function, disorganization of the body's energetic system which means that we are excessively cold, hot when we are not supposed to, etc. Nowadays, a warning indicating that cigarettes are harmful to our health, although the characters of these warnings can be seen only under microscope follows many advertisements for tobacco products.

Consequences Of Smoking

It is estimated that tobacco is costing Canadian and American families $ 10 billion a year (That was in 1990,today, it should be between 100 to 200 billions), because so many wage earners are dying soon. No matter from what angle we look at the smoking habits, we see nothing interesting, encouraging; only the trouble it is bound to bring to someone' s life one day. These troubles not only wean him from his fondness for life, but also may indeed even separate him from it. For me, tobacco is something we grow trying to justified death or something.

Yes, indeed, the danger of smoking tobacco, the troubles it creates in smokers' life are well known facts now, accepted by professionals as well as by the human in the street. Dr. Linus C. Pauling, twice a Nobel Prize winner, calculated that smoking 20 cigarettes a day diminishes life expectancy by 8 years, while smoking 40 cigarettes shortens the smokers' life by 26 years. So, as Sydney Petrie put it in his book," Make no mistake about it if you are still smoking, you are shortening your life expectancy; you are committing suicide the slow, hard way". No one knows why Rene Levesque died the way he did: suddenly, without a warning sickness. According to autopsy, it was heart failure. But everyone knows that he was a chain smoker. Certainly his smoking has something to do with his death, more especially so as he made a point of not seeing a doctor during his life. Now, many flight companies are banning cigarette smoking during their flights. Governments ban smoking in their buildings .All that has been done because everybody is convinced of the new fact that tobacco smoke in the confined air is as much a lethal weapon as smoking in general. They find that it causes lung cancer in people who don't smoke.

Another doctor, Leo Kimlen, conducted a research in London. Let's read the results: Where There is Smoke= Associated Press- Death from leukemia among heavy smokers was 50% higher than among non-smokers a study shows. The research published in the British Medical Journal showed that the leukemia death rate among people who smoke fewer than 10 cigarettes was 34% higher than the non -smokers. For cigarette smoker of 10 to 20 cigarettes a day, it was 57% higher, and for smokers of 20 or more, it was 63%, according to the study. 'If the findings in our study represents a direct relationship between smoking and leukemia, then it must follow that smoking is responsible for more cases of leukemia than all the hitherto-established causes combined' said the doctor .The study involved 248000 veterans from 1954 to 1969. During that period, 1723 died of leukemia. Of those 330 were smokers, 185 were ex-smokers, 46 smoke cigars, and 162 non-smokers! Province September 13,1988.

The necessity to kick away the habit is also illustrated, elsewhere, by Health and Welfare. Their figures showed that there were **35 000 deaths a year in Canada from tobacco smoke related diseases (1973)**

Even the court system in its own way has started to recognize the link between tobacco and some deadly diseases. This statement is well demonstrated by the case of Mrs. Rose Carillon who sued a cigarette company while she was dying of lung cancer. When she died, her husband pursued the law suit, lost in most courts, but was eventually awarded $ 400 000 against Ligett Group, which makes Chesterfield cigarettes. Another court case was won by relatives of a man who died after smoking Marlboro for 4 decades. Philip Morris was ordered to pay to that family $75.5 as punitive damage award in 1999 for knowingly keep secret the information that smoking is harmful to the body of the smoker. In the recent years court, life has been tumultuous, bombarded by law suits against tobacco products companies. Even governments jumped in the bandwagon, although, as I said above, they are agent of promotion of the usage of tobacco product, consequently agent of promotion of tobacco addiction, for not banning the culture of tobacco, for preferring tobacco $ taxes over the ban despite that the effects of smoking cost them more, when they are not selling it themselves. The existence of a country, among 190 countries, where tobacco product is sold by the state is imaginable.

Doctors are giving their patient's ultimatum to quit smoking, smoking is banned in public places in many countries and on public transportation, these are all signs that the habit of smoking is considered as a threat, a danger to our health and our life. Researchers help scientists and doctor establish a list of diseases related to smoking. As far as he is concerned, he thinks a lot more diseases are related to the habit of smoking unheard of. He think also AIDS and more sexual diseases may be related to that habit. What are you waiting for to kick it away?

Summarization of consequences of smoking:

- smoking and
- blindness
- infertility

- libido decrease
- stroke
- heart attack even before the age of 50
- lung cancer
- asthma
- fire hazard
- useless expenses to buy tobacco product

Among the points the points covered in this chapter were: unhealthy, deadly chemical elements found in tobacco smoke--Millions of death a year linked to smoking, -Some diseases related to smoking, established by many researches---The cost of the use of tobacco product on the tax payer is evaluated at billion $ a year in medical expenses--Doctors say cigarettes diminish life expectancy--Research established link between smoking and leukemia, etc.

Let's move on now to the last curious issue addressed in this work--- States tergiversation--- on the road to kick the habit away and install the appropriate psychological power to stay out of it all the times.

Chapter III

C) IF SMOKING ENDANGERS LIFE WHY DON'T STATES FORBID THE CULTURE OF TOBACCO AND THE SALE OF ITS PRODUCTS?

States don't forbid these things because they are hooks on tobacco taxes as hinted in the previous chapter. The problem is not as simple as it sounds. Human lives are involved in the two opposite sides of the issue. Seeing it from one side, people are dying because diseases related to smoking. Seeing it from the other side, the well being of many persons is dependent on the sale of tobacco. That is to say there are workers in the industry with families to take care of, to feed. Governments would have to take sides to solve the problem once and for all. Anyway, they prefer not to make a decision on it. And the indecision itself creates a sort of side effect problem for the tobacco farmers. This is David Ramer the grower you see in the picture says in relation to that:" The indecision is killing us. The outlook is so uncertain, we don't have our heart in the business. It is demoralizing and we no longer have the capital to lunch another business"(The Financial Post, June 20th, 1988,pp 41,42). It is no good anymore to be in that business. Unless tobacco could be converted to another product, another use (They found that it could be transformed in protein with no hazardous effect in Cuba).

Prosperity comes to an end for Ontario growers

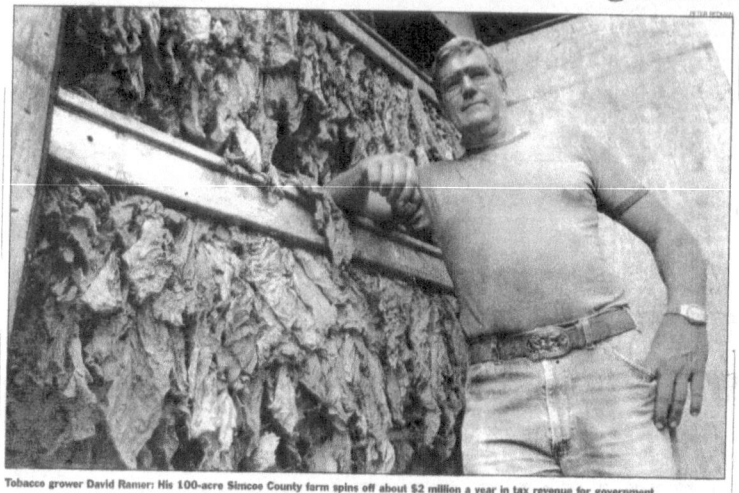

Tobacco grower David Ramer: His 100-acre Simcoe County farm spins off about $2 million a year in tax revenue for government

Smoking tobacco is definitely a killing habit that we can spare. It would be better for us all if governments decided to banish the culture of tobacco for smoking once and for all instead of leaving the tobacco farmers up in the air, in agony.

Cultivating tobacco can also become addictive, for it yields better results than almost anything else. Here is what France Phillips of the Financial Post had to say on that:" Although, raw tobacco prices have not increased beyond our average $ 1.70 a pound in 4 years, tobacco still provides for farmers better returns than just about any crop on earth". Typically, tobacco grosses a farmer $ 4, 000.00 an acre. Prairie farmers count themselves lucky if they gross $ 175.00 per acre from wheat. Field tomatoes gross about $ 2200.00 an acre, peanuts $750.00 per acre.

Several Ontario farmers were experimenting with ginseng, purportedly a cure for a variety of ailments including impotence. Although, the root sells for $ 60-100 a pound in Asia, growers must invest $ 50 0000.00 over 4 years before reaping a harvest. And it is a rot-prone crop.' There is no quick fix or magic crop' laments Arthur Lougthon, manager of Ontario Ministry of Agriculture and Food Transition Team.

The role of tobacco in economic structure of countries such as Canada,

United States, Zimbabwe, probably Cuba (etc.), is very significant, for it concerned the biggest producers of tobacco in the world, for Canada and United States, a multibillion $ industry. In the young People and Smoking Arthur Cain wrote" Where tobacco, for example spinach, it would have been prohibited and thrown out years ago without any controversy. But you can't do that with a multibillion $ industry". All in all, the production of tobacco puts $ 3.3 billion in the coffer of the treasury of United States each year. So many Americans are reluctant to give up what procures them work and higher standard of living.

The author of kickitwell still disagrees with the fellow Americans on this point. If there were a comparative study in United States, to find how much growing tobacco provides society with in terms of money from taxes and how much it destroys, I am sure it would be clear that it destroys much more than it provides. Treating people sick from smoking tobacco products (If they didn't inhale they wouldn't be sick, may be; they do inhale despite what a certain Tonclin has said once) is expensive. Workdays lost, all that cost all taxpayers a bundle, a lot of money.

In British Columbia with a population of 4,249,253(1999 census), $468 million were collected last year, 2001,in tax revenue on tobacco products. The same year, $1.6 billion were spent to cure tobacco related illness. So the deficit in this category was more than one billion. All Canada together that's about 7 billion deficit. In regard to United States, the deficit was roughly $98billion.In other words, if these governments banish the culture of tobacco, they would save billions of dollars, lot of dough that could be used partly to help transforming tobacco farmers into farmers of something else.

Then, there is more in the explanation of the indecision on banishing the sale of tobacco products. The sellers of these products have big muscles in terms of finance. They can toss away another person just like that, even persons of governments. Remember how Prime Minister Jean Chretien tossed away that guy activist who was a threat for the Prime Minister life during a protestation. The financial giants in the tobacco industry can do it just like that with their opponents. Here is a story I have read in The Province: The airline company Northwest 800 banned tobacco smoking in all its flights. The tobacco lobby sets its computers telling all its addicted friends to call the airline number and talk about its poor 'On time performance' and 132 violations of the Federal Aviation Standard. Anyway, those actions by the industry demonstrates well why your governments don't help you in kicking the habit away by not banishing the culture of tobacco and the sale of tobacco products. And, because governments don't banish the culture of tobacco for sale once and for all doesn't mean it is not a killing undertaking.

Why then it is not banished once and for all? Governing personalities have this information. Democracy is responsible for this state of thing, it's like. No political party wants to jeopardize its time in power by making a drastic move in banishing the culture of tobacco. The issue is too hot I guess.

Some of the important ideas in this chapter were:

1. Governments are hooks on the so-called "Sin taxes".

2. It would be better if governments banish the culture of tobacco for smoking once and for all.

3. Cultivating tobacco yields better results than almost any thing else in terms of profit for farmers.

4. Governments would save lot of dough by banishing the culture of tobacco for smoking, money that could be used partly to help tobacco farmers transforming into farmers of something else.

Despite the recognition that the habit is a threat to life, an important number of you are still puffing. Is it because it's so difficult to kick the habit far away from you or because you are not using your inherent power efficiently enough yet? Let's move on the next issue to find out.

Chapter IV

D) WHAT MAY MAKE IT NOT EASY TO KICK IT AWAY ON YOUR OWN?

The "creator" of this method avoids talking to his friends about tobacco, because they have tried to quit smoking unsuccessfully. You don't want to make someone feel embarrassed or something. Many people stop puffing many times. Why is it such difficult thing to do, to stop sucking tobacco smoke without some professional help? Why do intelligent people (I am so I think instead of I think so I am) keep smoking against their will, in face of mountains of evidence that it is a harmful habit?

The answer to these questions is not a clear- cut matter either, for there might be as many reasons not to kick the habit away, as there are individuals.

Despite the irreducible aspects of the questions above I am going to attempt to provide you with a coherent answer. First of all, it's a lack of opportunity to know about habit formation/deformation and how the mind works what would allow you to control the major tri-ggers

And get rid of any unwanted habit. He already said that in traditional and alternative medicine it is not clear that the mind is understood for what it is a non-substantial reality. It gets mixed up with the brain a substantial reality. If the nature of the mind is not understood, let alone how it functions; if health professionals (physician and psychiatrist) not always understand, acknowledge or taking into account in health practices that the mind is not physical, let alone people in other fields of work, in the street.

Second of all, the same way you started to smoke inadvertently, the same way you continue. Some of you started it because it is an adult thing to do or because it's one way you choose to demonstrate your masculinity, manhood, even freedom to decide for yourself what to do or not. Some of you smoke because you want to show to the rest of the world, to your friends, that your are modern non- prude, a good sport.

Third of all, there is Sydney Petrie in How to Quit Smoking in Three Days who has a more colorful explanation for you. According to him, people don't kick the habit away because they are thumb suckers, pencil chewers, toothpick eaters, similarly engaging in the mechanism of substitution. Still according to him, there are the retaliation smoker, the handling smoker, the craving smoker and the stimulation smoker.

Although these sub-types are all defined by their names, the author of Kickitwell is going to expand on them in order to explain the process a bit. The Crutch Smoker looks like someone who leans on cigarette or cigar or pipe as a crutch when under a stressful situation. The food faddist exchanges fat for nicotine at cellular level. Even that is wrong. **Research find that men who smoke may weigh less, however, more of their body fat is deposited around the waist in a spare tire pattern, linked to a higher risk of heart disease, diabetes and premature death**. The retaliation smoker is obviously in a state of rebellion. The stimulating smoker wakes his mind up with the chemical element contained in tobacco products without paying too much attention of what he/she is doing to his/her body and his/her health.

Not kicking the habit away for retaliation seems to be fundamental in the personality of all unable to quitters, especially the young ones. Most of them don't kick the habit away because they don't accept the interdiction that makes smoking appear "sinful" and cigarette "the product of the devil itself". Deeply, they are saying that a simple tobacco product doesn't have such power. They are right.

Fourth of all, some of you may use smoking as socializing means, or as a way to meet the opposite sex. It's like it would be easier to break the ice between 2 strangers or 2 sexes by asking or offering cigarette or matches. If you don't want to give up the habit, then it's ok, but if you want to kick it away the socializing factor cannot be an excuse, for there are many other ways to socialize and meet the other half.

Fifth of all, the tobacco industry may keep you puffing through subliminal advertisement. We are on a slippery ground, nevertheless, during the last United States election, there was an ad sponsored by the republican side in which Mr. Gore was subliminally qualified as being a rat. You all know the result of that election. Mr. Gore wasn't elected. Was the subliminal message effective? Not easy to say, but the result allows us to think it was. So too can subliminal ads prevent you from giving up the lung cancer prone habit.

Sixth of all, Michael A.H. Russell of the Addiction Research Unit, Manley Hospital, London, says that a steady, heavy smoker seeks to avoid the pain of nicotine withdrawal, whereas a light smoker is keeping the habit for kicks.

Let's go to the last sub-part of this issue, some statements, which have frequently been given as reasons why a person continues to smoke. Avram Goldstein first published them, M.D. in Learn More Smoke Free. They're 18, I would like you to find yourself pencil and comment on each one of them in the blank space, then compare your comment with mine in the next page. Some of you may find your comments much more brilliant than mine that will be ok.

1. The relationship between smoking and cancer has not really been proven.

   _____

   _____

   _____

   _____

2. Smoking won't shorten my life by more than 5 years, and it's better to enjoy life now than to live five years longer and be unhappy.

_____

_____

_____

_____

3. I have been smoking so long that the damage has already been done.

_____

_____

_____

_____

4. I am truly addicted therefore unable to stop.

_____

_____

_____

_____

5. We don't stop the used of alcohol and automobile, yet they are more dangerous than cigarettes.

_____

_____

_____

_____

6. I have to smoke to relieve my nerves.

_____

_____

_____

_____

7. I smoke filter tips; the harmful material has been largely removed.

_____

_____

_____

_____

8. When I stop smoking I gain weight and that's just as bad.

_____

_____

_____

_____

9. Anything (including cigarettes) is good in moderation bad in excess.

_____

_____

_____

_____

10. I personally know at least one very old person who has smoked most of his life yet continues to be in fine health. There is no cancer in my family, so therefore I need not to worry much about it.

_____

_____

_____

_____

11. Cancer comes with age and heredity. There is no cancer in my family; therefore I need not to worry much about it.

_____

_____

_____

_____

12. Hydrogen bomb, highway accidents, murders, alcoholism, suicide-so there is no safety anywhere- why worries about it?.

_____

_____

_____

_____

13. The pleasure I get, which is certain, outweighs the health hazard, which is uncertain.

_____

_____

_____

_____

14. The emotional effect of my going without cigarettes is more hazardous to me than smoking.

_____

_____

_____

_____

15. Scientific research will develop 'safe' cigarettes before too long, and the effect of my smoking between now and then is probably insignificant.

_____

_____

_____

_____

16. Under present conditions, who wants to live long?.

_____

_____

_____

_____

17. God would not have tobacco plant on earth if he didn't have a non-harmful purpose in mind.

_____
_____
_____
_____

18. Smoking proves I am weak-willed. Everybody is entitled to one weakness.

_____
_____
_____
_____

My comments are of diverse backgrounds. It can be very hard and very tormenting for someone who wants to kick it away and not being able to do so. Not knowing the little principle: habit formation/deformation, not knowing how the mind works, how to control the habit triggers, (the only way to be 100% sure you really quit despite tons of gadgets that may or may not help) people delude themselves into these rationalizations. I am going to comment only on the statements ,not on the people who made them. It good exercise for you who want to kick it away. It will allow you to think of more of the problematic, which, in turn, will help you to quit. So here we go:

1. This statement might have been made in 1980, when the evidence relating smoking and cancer was not gathered, convincing and publicized as it is now in 2002. How about the newspaper titles .n this work?

2. People who never smoke don't miss nicotine.

3. Better late than never. Please, read again introduction of Remedy. Besides, most parts of the body renew themselves completely

many times during the course of a life. So if you kick it away, your brand new lung will have nothing to do with it.

4. Because addiction is an acquired habit it can be eliminated. Please, read again the introduction of Remedy.

5. Automobiles help cross miles in winter in a relatively short period of time. Tobacco smoke helps with nothing real, concrete.

6. Read a book on how to cope with stress or stress management.

7. I think filter tips serve only big companies that sell cigarettes.

8. There are a lot of weight control programs available.

9. Yes, except that it is addictive and that in this context moderation is not easy.

10. First, we cannot know for sure how fine a person is health wise, if we haven't read her medical file. Second, everybody does not react to the same chemical substance the same way at the same time. I mean by that the bad news might have been only postponed. Third, a whole lot of sicknesses are mentioned in chapter How Smoking Endangers Life, more, there other types of effects such as burning your house and/or yourself falling asleep while indulging in the habit.

11. The bad effect of tobacco smoke in our body is related to cancer, but also to other diseases such as, heart stroke, gangrene, etc.

12. It's like saying:" I am already sick in one foot, why worry about the other?" Also, population growth is a fact, then alter the concern about accident, murders, alcoholism and suicide.

13. What pleasure could we get from nicotine?

14. The mind that makes you sick can also heal you. Relax, trust

yourself. 5 minutes turmoil is worth a life of freedom. How do you know if you haven't try?

15. Researchers are not interested in safe cigarette. They are interested in curing cancer. Big tobacco product companies are not interested in safe cigarettes either. They are interested in making profit. Governments: How are we going to do to win the next election? How about taxes? So you are really left with yourself to solve the problem, all problems as a matter of fact

16. Is it possible to live in a vacuum? The puzzle is part of the deal. Life is like that. You must always be solving a new problem. There is no need to lose hope, especially equipped with a mind such as ours. We will have most of the important answers. But for that to happen, an attitude of optimism is required. We have problem because we have the tool to solve them. Problem is disharmony with self. As you have already guessed : solution is harmony with self.

17. That non-harmful purpose of God might not necessarily be smoking tobacco product. Besides, God had never created the tobacco we smoke. The tobacco that we smoke is a man made product through hybridization of natural products similar to tobacco.

18. Everybody is also entitled to good health, sheer pleasure of living and long life.Please, read Psycho synthesis written by Roberto Assagioli. There is a part on how to train your will.

Summarization:

Cigarettes symbolize many things for you; retaliation; avoiding pain or you continue the habit for kicks ,etc.

You keep puffing for many reasons. Here are some of them; lack of opportunity to know what addiction really is, about habit formation/deformation etc. The would allow you to control the majors triggers and get rid of any kind of toxic habit or addiction .In other words, you weren't able to quit on your own because you didn't take it seriously enough weren't convinced enough of the danger in smoking, hope picture below help you achieving that, you didn't focus on yourself and on give it up enough .

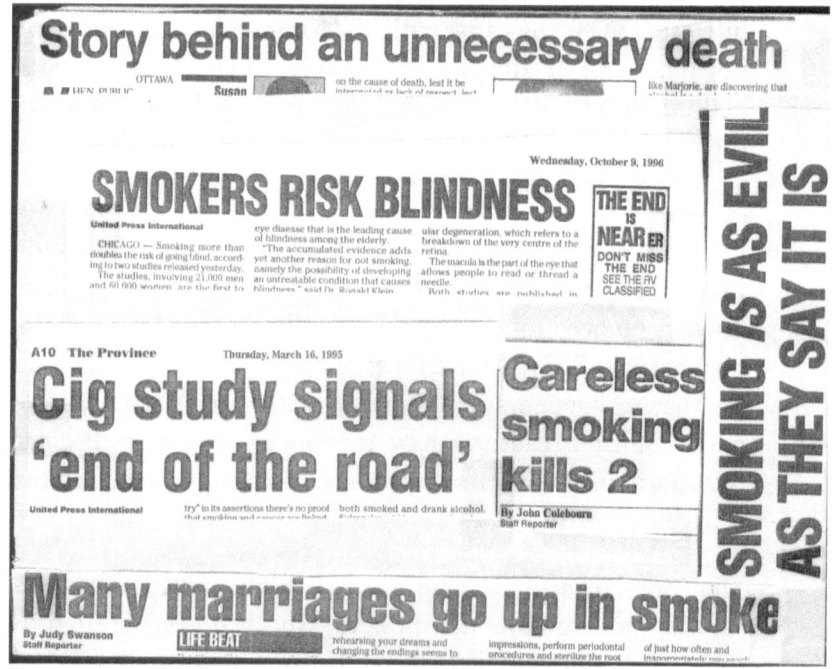

Part of the title is KICKITWELLORELSE, suggesting that there is the proper way, the right means at everyone disposal ,to give up any unwanted habit. In the next part of this work, I'll show you how to do that. Let's move on to it.

PART II

Remedy

Whenever we want to change some of our habits, there will be a number of factors that enhance or assist the implementation. There will also be a number of factors or events inhibiting the change.

J. Burton Cunningham Ph. D.

Drug hardly ever appeal to people involved in something that matters to them.

Robert Fritz

Chapter V

A LITTLE BIT OF HISTORY

Some of you who want to give up the habit and don't succeed yet may rationalize that if it was such a bad thing to do, nature wouldn't create tobacco in the first place. Actually, this sort of rationalization is in the mind of everybody, for it appears to make sense. Nonetheless, here is the hiccup. The tobacco that some of you have been smoking has never been found in nature. In other words, the smoking tobacco is "man" made product by hybridization. It is stated clearly in the book named "Tobacco" written by B.C. Akehurst in the following:" Nicotiana tabacum is an amphidiploids which has never been found in the truly wild state. Its uniquely high proportion in alkaloids occurring as nicotine has led Dawson(1960) to consider that its survival as a species is due entirely to "man" protection. The creation of new species and the formation of new amphidiploids are recognized botanical occurrence".

ADDICTION DEFINITION AND PRINCIPLES INVOLVED

DEFINITION-

1) NEW OXFORD: **a fact or condition of being addicted to a particular substance, thing or activity;**

2) UNABRIDGED RANDOM HOUSE: **state of being enslaved to a habit or practice or something that psychologically, physically**

habit forming as narcotic to such an extent that its cessation leaves severe trauma.

Principles Involved

These definitions are incomplete, for one thing there is no trauma to be left, if the cessation is done properly. Nonetheless, they let us guess that there is something powerful to cause the inability to kick the habit away without a fuss. In other words it's about **psychological power.** When you were a smoker of cigarettes, and didn't want to quit, after a certain time it became a psychological power according to this equation:

voluntary acts>> habit>> psychological power(voluntary acts, then habit, then psychological power).

When you want to quit and unable to do so sometimes, it is because of the previous formation of the psychological power, but now it becomes a problem. That is why we have to add a third definition of **addiction: an unwanted psychological power.**

It is not accepted, as welcome as it was before. We can't give up the habit, because the first reaction is to attack the psychological power which is like attacking nature, like wanting to catch a fish by its tail. We will not succeed there.

The equation above is what the author called **habit formation principle.**

Then we have another principle which is **habit deformation**

Which is obtained by multiplying the act by 0 what gives us the second equation:

0 act>0 habit>0 power, in other words no act, no habit, no power

Seen in this context, it is not as difficult to get rid of addiction. To do so we only have to reverse the formation process of the psychological power.

Psychological power means that part of the act becomes unconscious, you do it without having to think of it very much. The unconscious takes care of it. The same is true in the deformation process. After a while, the unconscious takes charge and cancels the many triggers you will not even be able to think of let alone control.

Then anyone can quit using this method because of what we have seen, also because every single person is intelligent, has formed and cancelled many psychological powers in a life time many psychological powers in a life time.

In a way, we can say memory doesn't like the new, for memory exists to keep humanly events, like a stock- keeper, in the mind. Its function is rather conservative, more related to the past. When we try to put something new in it, it rejects it at first. The question is something is new for how long? So the rejection will not last. In that sense, you are addicted for being unaware of little facts such as this about memory and the mind and the psyche. **Addiction to smoking is memory going ashtray,** another possible definition definition.

Like flottable in water, memory of addiction needs energy at first to stay at the bottom of the mind and so being somewhat deactivated. It is also something to be handled carefully. For after a while you have to let it go, let the unconscious system takes it over. Anyway, it will be impossible for you to prevent it from rising to the surface of the mind for sometime, until its energy is diminished enough to keep it away from you.

Even after being inactivated, it (the urge to indulge) will rise up and sink back as quickly, if it's not in your expectation.

So, after you get rid of the habit, if you compulsively think of it, or see it in your dream, it's not that the method you have used is not effective, not a sign you are not succeeding. It is in the nature of things.

Then comes the concept of **trigger. After the voluntary act is made a number of times in a context, the context becomes a trigger of that act, for example, after you smoke a number of times while having a meal, meals become a trigger of smoking, meaning that they create the urge to smoke.** There can be so many triggers in a smoker's life, we can forget about the idea of controlling them all. To be able to get rid of the habit it is sufficient to control only the major ones.

Further- more, some triggers are more powerful than others are. People smoke a cigarette immediately before or after or after making love. People smoke also while having a cup of coffee. It is obvious the coffee trigger is very much less powerful than the love making one. Therefore, it is necessary to pay attention to the more powerful triggers too.

So the method I am proposing to you to help kick the habit (any habit with adaptation) away is based on these psychological principles . It goes this way:

Step I—Preparation

a) Read KICKITWELL booklet entirely and understand it.

b) Get rid of all tobacco products: cigarettes, cigars, ashtrays etc.

c) Stop the habit.

d) Take it easy. If you can tell yourself a joke before each exercise, go for it. The attitude is a playful one.

e) Remember this: Giving up addiction by using a psychological method such as this one requires 10% action, 90% of motivation and attitude.

f) When big stress is possible, such as break-ups, divorced, lost of job, death of family member, it is not the best time to do it. Postpone the quitting project until you are distress free or when it si quieter in that sense. There are lot of books on how to cope and get rid of ditress. I write about that in TIPS K at the end of this work.

Step II—Find The Triggers Of The Habit

1) Find out the occasions that trigger the habit. In general, they are joyful situations, stressful situations. Do you indulge in it before during

or after a meal? What other situations in your individual life you have associated with it making those situations prompting the habit? Make a list of the major and most powerful ones.

2) Devise strategies to control the triggers you have found in order to counteract, cancel or deviate their trigging function. Write down what you are going to do in order not to indulging in the habit around your next meal, your traditional cup of coffee or if you will simply keep away from smoking ?

STEP III—VISUALIZE YOURSELF FREE OF IT

1) Visualize yourself in situations free of the habit, until you are sure you are not coming back at it, that it was something you did in the past.

You already have a list of triggers. Use it for this exercise. See yourself in your imagination eating without smoking, asking someone out without having a cigarette in your hand, learning you have won millions of dollars without having to do it, drinking coffee without it. See yourself in all situations without indulging in the habit. Visualize doing something different :chewing gum talking to a friend instead if you want, or simply be. Do the exercise with each trigger you have written down on your list(not abslutly necessary) each day for 15 minutes during the quitting process.

It is an easy but still a powerful little exercise. Everyone knows how powerful imagination is. Anyone can quit this habit or any habit as a matter of fact just by it.

2) Reinforce the free image of yourself by:

    a)   going to support meetings. Some of them are free of charge and organized by governments, Narcotic Anonymous, 604 873 1018, in Vancouver, for example. You can even start your own group of support for ex-smokers through the Internet and indulge in the deliberation, in ideas that you can solve all the problems of the world, instead of smoking or letting yourself invaded by any unwanted habit.

b) engaging in creative activities.

2 to cancel if you are already a busy person.

STEP IV—SELF DIRECTION

Who said:" You can't teach a person anything, you can only help them find it within themselves." Galileo Galilei

And who said "No one can be healed against his will" Jane Roberts

Ask your self, higher self(will is closest to it) that is, to help you in the process of kicking it away. Notice the answers during your dream. your relaxed state, meditation or in what your feelings. Do whatever is suggested, if you understand. If not just do the asking for 5 minutes every day during the quitting process.

STEP V—COUNTERACTING RELAPSES

Controlling urges is something you do using your rational mind rather than your feelings.

Two ways to counteract relapses:

1. You ignore them and continue applying the steps as if they didn't happen, until they don't happen or

2. Post a blank sheet of paper on the wall of your office or at home (with 2 empty columns one for date and the other for circumstances). Each time you relapse, write down date and circumstances in which the relapsing occurred.

The ideal is you will write on this paper once or twice or even not at all, but no matter what happened continue the application of 2 until you give up the habit. In other words don't let them fool you into believing that you can't quit.

Which ever the way you choose to control relapses, why don't use the repressed energy to

a) Do physical conditioning: cardiovascular, flexing, and strength exercise;

b) Loose wait or whatever you wanted to do to have a better life but never had the opportunity to do before this time.

Chapter VI

THE TIPS TO HELP YOU
KICK IT AWAY FASTER

A) Tips For Family and Friends

This one was going to be forgotten . I put it first in this writing among the other tips to emphasize its importance. For, one person told me once" I didn't quit smoking using your method because my wife made me smoke when she thought that I was in some sort of a struggle. A journalist wrote this tip. Here it is:

- Quitting smoking is genuinely hard. Be sympathetic and supportive--
- Don't judge and don't nag!
- The new ex-smoker will likely have weird emotions and feelings. Bear with them.
- Most important: All smokers and quitters are different and only they know the best things you can do to help them. They might want company, for example, or to be left alone. Ask first And, as one team member says above, don't take any of it personally.

B) Self-Hypnosis

Hypnosis is usually thought of as an inter- personal relationship in which one individual (the hypnotist) gives directions or suggestions to another individual the (subject). This is termed as" hetero-hypnosis". There is, however, another way the person can reach the hypnotic state. This involves only one person, the subject, and his own "autohypnosis" or self -hypnosis. In this case a person learns to give himself the directions necessary to achieve the hypnotic state and when in it to provide the suggestions that will work for his benefit. It can be effective as hetero-hypnosis, and in some cases even more effective, since there is little reason a person should feel motivated to resist a suggestion he himself puts forth.

Pavlov's theory of conditioning is particularly useful when apply to learning self-hypnosis. A sound, a light, even a thought can be the stimulus, the trigger, to produce a particular response or behavior leading to an hypnotic state is that the subject is able to accept suggestion that he wouldn't otherwise, in a normal waking state, accept and then to benefit from those suggestions. So, if you feel you might give self-hypnotism a try, to help get rid of those cigarettes, safely, comfortably, and permanently, I suggest you read on. With a bit of practice on one of the techniques set forth here, you can do just that - stop smoking safely, comfortably and permanently

To begin you should read through the following procedures to familiarize yourself with the ideas outlined. It is not necessary to memorize the words; just recognize the responses that are to be produced by stimuli or triggers, then find yourself a very comfortable chair where you can prop your feet up, or lie down on a couch, provide as distraction -free an environment as possible, and begin to practice the trigger or signal with a desired response. After enough repetition of the procedure the trigger will produce the behavior response automatically. Here then is one method.

Now for the trigger or signal I want you to use the word R-E-L-A-X.

1.   Begin by thinking of the first R. as you do, I want you to begin to relax and to formulate suggestion with regard to how long you want to stay in the hypnotic state. You know what time it is now when you are beginning. Decide on a time when you want to "wake up" from your hypnotic state- maybe 15 minutes from now. Think of the letter R, begin to relax, and think of

the time now, and then decide on the time you wish to awaken! Isn't this easy so far?

2. E stands for entering the hypnotic state. Think of E, while beginning to experience also heaviness in your eyelids, as if your eyes wanted to close. Concentrate on the letter E and begin to be aware of tiredness and fatigue in your eyes and of how much more comfortable they would be if you just allow them to close. E stands for entering the hypnotic state, allowing your weary eyes to close, going to "sleep".

3. L will be the signal to loosen up, both physically and mentally. I mean to let yourself go and just allow the chair to support you as if you were a big rag dull. Loosen up! To aid you in feeling this loosening, I want you to concentrate in kind of progressive relaxation. Begin by relaxing all the muscles in your feet; let them go very limp and loose. Then allow this feeling to drift up to your ankles, into your calves and your knees- just a feeling of limp, loose heaviness- and from your knees it will ascend to your thighs and your abdomen. Let the muscles go very loose and slack. Now allow the feeling to move upward into chest and your shoulders, your arms and your hands. Let them relax, limp and slack. Even the muscles of your neck can experience this looseness, this wonderful, comfortable relaxation. Let the small muscles of your face go loose. All your body can experience this feeling of loosening up!

4. Visualize A. It sands for advance deepening. You are very relax now, but you can relax even more deeply, go into even a more relax and comfortable state. Help yourself to reach deeper stages of relaxation by counting backwards from 5 down to 1. In your mind, see and hear and think of going into a deeper and deeper relaxed state, stepping down into deeper and deeper stages of relaxation; at five, let go more and more, drifting deeper and deeper into relaxation; at four, become looser, limper, and more and more slack, a big limp rag doll. At three, sink deeper and deeper into the chair, more nearly like being asleep. At two, all your body continuing to relax more and more, drifting lower,

deeper, closer to sleep. When you think of one, you will be in a very, very deep sleep, soundly asleep. Your thoughts are completely relaxed, deeply relaxed and you are in a very deep sleep, a deep, comfortable, satisfying sleep. Tell yourself: If for any reason I should need to awaken before the time I have decided on, I will be able to do so immediately, capable of doing whatever I need to do. Deeply asleep now, deeply relaxed.

Visualize X. it is the symbol for being in a state of extra suggestibility. Because of your deep relaxation, your mind is free to accept the suggestions you will provide. Because of the deep state of relaxation you are in, your mind will completely "soak up" the suggestions you have prepared for it, and you will continue to be affected by the suggestions even when you are no longer in the trance-state and extra suggestible -highly responsive to your own suggestions which will so greatly benefit you. At the signal X, you will think of the suggestions you have prepared for yourself. When you first begin the technique, you will give yourself neutral suggestions that are easy for you to accept so that you will cause no anxiety to interfere with your hypnotic relaxation. Say to yourself "next time I practice the procedure I will be able to relax even more deeply and even more quickly" and "I will be able to clear my mind to respond more easily to the suggestions I will give, and the suggestion will always be very- very effective" Once you have conditioned yourself to the hypnotic state by numerous repetitions of the above procedure, one right after the other, you will be ready to proceed to give yourself suggestions related to helping you to stop smoking (Sydney Petrie).

C) Psychic Ability Development

There is an even more potent technique than hypnosis to acquire an ability, discovered by the author of kickitwell who calls it psychic ability development .It is in two steps, simpler but may be less easy to do than hypnotism. Here it is:

1. Before going to bed, you write down ability you want to acquire,

leaving a space beside to write it in the morning. Example "I will be able to strengthen my will to kick it away soon".

In the morning, you write down your dream, find the part that corresponds to the ability, write it in the space left for this purpose. It may be not in clear terms, you might have to interpret it; but you will recognize it.

D) THE INTENSITY OF THE CRAVING LASTS VERY LITTLE TIME.

After a few minutes or so it starts to decrease. So if you can go through these few minutes without inhaling, you win a battle. In other words, in a longer-term basis you will win the war against this habit you come to despise, if you keep at it.

E) GENEROSITY IS HELPFUL FOR YOUR OWN LIBERATION, IN THAT IT TEACHES YOU ABOUT THE INNER QUALITY OF LETTING GO.

Letting go and releasing your attachment are the most freeing things you can do to liberate yourself from the ego. A need to hang on into things and money that you received arises out an inner sense of incompleteness. Practicing generosity aligns you with your sense of completeness" and may help you kick it away.

F) GIVING UP SOMETHING CAN BE A HARD THING TO DO EVEN IF IT'S NOT A GOOD THING YOU ARE GIVING UP.

It's a put down to your acquisitive instinct. Your cognitive system must undergo a series of transformations trying to fill up the emptiness left by what your body considered to have lost. While this inner "brassage" is taking place our personality structure, our personhood may be shaken. We may become "very sensitive, emotional, a bombshell". Despite all that, nevertheless, you had given things up, you are giving things up, and will give things up all the time. Sometimes it may be conscious as when we give up old cloths, pieces of furniture, cars, even friends, things we feel we no longer need, things we find unnecessary, annoying. The giving up can also be unconscious as when we comb our hair, cleaning up or going to the toilet. So **giving things up is among the fundamental principles of life. Kick it away is nothing unusual.**

G) DARE YOURSELF NOT TO TOUCH A CIGARETTE AGAIN.

After a few non fruitful trials, one day he woke up mad, leaving the half full package of Dumaurier on the coffee table and dare himself not to touch it again, in his apartment in a building at the corner of Davie and Broughton. Since this moment, the habit becomes something of the past, has been put off indefinitely. When we don't want to do something, there is no power left in it. We may continue to act automatically governed by stimuli in our environment. But with firm resolution even the unnatural environment can't make you do something you don't want to do. That is one conclusion of the way he quit.

The half-full package of Dumaurier was in front of his eyes for sometime, but the habit was kicked away for good. It was like taking the bull by the horns. In other words, when you want to quit you don't, you are overwhelmed by the fear that you can't do it. When you do the fear is gone, another conclusion.

H) BENEFITS IN KICKING AWAY THE HABIT

The benefits we can gain from kicking it away are of various categories. Oral hygiene must come first to mind when thinking of benefits there are in kicking it away You will have clean bright white teeth. Next, we may think of cleanliness of our body, fingers without stains, clear skinned complexion. If you drive and smoke your shirts may have hole in them after some cigarette's sparks have been blown on them by the wind. The same way the back seat may have holes in it also.

Many houses burst into flames because of smoking.

Those are among few of the visible benefits there is in kicking it away, for not having to deal with these negative consequences: money to buy new shirts. the replace the back seat of your car, etc.

But there are invisible benefits too.

Our tastes change for the better.

We feel livelier. That is exactly what happens after kicking it away. We feel as if our senses come to life after a long hibernation. Remember that smoke is able to penetrate the deepest part of our body, all its tiny fibers putting our senses in a sort of lethargic state. Kicking it away is like a rejuvenation process.

Those bring us to a little story .It was around 8 o'clock in the morning, very nice out. The sun was majestically perched on the horizon of a clear blue sky. I came off the sky Train at 22nd Street in New Westminster, going to catch a connecting bus to get me to work, teacher on call at Delta. While waiting for the bus, saw a beautiful young lady sitting on a bench waiting for the same bus. As I saw a smile hovered over her lips. She guessed I was admiring her beauty, she was right Those days when you feel making love would be pale, but only eating the woman would be satisfying although I would never hart any woman, let alone the one who attracts me so much. I started a little chat with her. . In the middle of our conversation, I noticed she was shivering. That was a surprise to me, given the fact that we were at the end of spring and it was not cold. Later on the same day, thinking back to the way she was shivering, and trying to find an explanation, I remember that she had a lighted cigarette between her fingers the whole time we were talking. It's like the smoke has mixed up her senses, particularly temperature sense perception, as written in chapter How Smoking Endangers Life. Of course when you kick it away it's no longer a problem, on the contrary, it's a benefit, too.

When you kick the habit away, your health is better, your sleep more restful so that you may need less of it. You will not cough without having a cold. Your general appearance is healthier so you are more appealing to the opposite sex. Etc.

I) Please Stop smoking before it's Too Late

"The main reasons I am speaking out on this subject is because of a note, my mother who is a heavy smoker, left in my room when she discovered that I smoke."

"She didn't yell or lecture me; she just left a note for me to think about. Thanks to her, I realized that endangering your life is not only stupid; it is avoidable, and if there are other women out there who care as much as mine did, many teens would learn a valuable lesson. Here is mom letter:

> Dear Sue: As a person, who is addicted to cigarettes, I would like to stop, but I am powerless to do so. Please stop smoking before it's too late!
>
> Your dad will bury me because smoking does shorten one's life. Did you ever take a look at my face? I look much older than I should at my age, and I can thank cigarette for this! I am not writing this as your mother, but as a cigarette smoker who knows the habit starts with one cigarette at a time--- then you get hooked and can't do anything about it.
>
> Love, Mom

Abby, please print my Mom's letter. May be someone else will realize that life is too precious to throw away and quit smoking.

Sue Duffy"

J) Advertisement for tobacco products embellishes indulgence in the habit.

Looking at the picture of an advertisement for tobacco product is like looking at a piece of paradise on earth. In these pictures usually there are the nicest choice of color and scenery, healthy and very good-looking people as suggested in this picture. The ideas in these ads convey appeal, always leaving in our mind a sense of well being. Despite the little warning, most of the time invisible, incomprehensible for the ordinary person, these advertisements leave us no choice of decision in our own lives. Smoking adults have less of a chance to resist the temptation than someone who has never indulged in the habit does. A young person has no chance at all.

"Teen age girls are most vulnerable to the influences in movies, on TV, and in fashion magazines"." The image of thinness that cigarettes promote, because they're thought to suppress appetite is not the only pressure. They also want to look older than they really are."Beauty program counters manufactured image by talking about real sources of attractiveness such as confidence, grace strength, humor, independence, and grooming" Joanna Ashworth, program for teen age girls Beauty From the Inside Out, in Manitoba, tel: 9836710.

Instead of the ugly effects of smoking, most of the time in the advertisement we find the most human preoccupations, human themes that are very dear to all of us such as the beauty of people, the comfort of the living room, sheer joy that cigarette supposed to provide us with, the adventurer, the cowboy, the party people, people who like flirting, and the sheer pleasure of smoking.

The woman above looks the way women do after making love, but she is just absorbing nicotine.The one on the bicycle below supposed to be extra sweet, living the here and now type of life, sport- pro, because she is a smoker, or because she is smoking this brand of cigarette. That is an illusion.

But beside the pack of cigarettes, if you saw Wayne Greasy and/or Michael Jordan and/or Venus William (I wish them the best, they would live 120 years or even more in the same shape they are now) in a wheelchair and if there was this message: "This product is carcinogenic and toxic, causes death and illness from cancer, heart disease and burger's disease- which leads to leg amputation- This product is addictive. Almost everybody would turn his or her head away after seeing such a product. Then, it would be easier to convince you not to start smoking.

There is this strange story about the paragraph above. It was first conceived in the 90s when, being dismissed from teaching and trying to create something to do beside researching, I wrote the first version of kickitwell. The new version started in January 2002. It was a surprise for me to hear and see in the news that Queen Elizabeth, during her recent visit to Vancouver asked to go and throw the first puck at hockey game(October 6, 2002), and insisted to be accompanied by Wayne Gretski to walk on the red carpet. Then the day after there was a Korean woman in a wheelchair who met her at Hotel Vancouver.

I would never think of putting queen Elizabeth and the woman in the wheelchair in the same picture.'

It's a bizarre event, for I am trying to create many things without success yet. Things I would never thought of creating are already done.

J) Researcher shows how ads fool people.

K) Stress and Quitting the Habit

You have already read the highest events during which you should not try to give up the habit in the steps. Anyway you might be experiencing an unusual amount of stress for reason only you know. Some thinking systems are stressful, because some of the pieces don't fit, because they are generated by irrational beliefs. Some theories, like the one according to which the world is seen as jungle in the introduction and forewords of this work, are stressful. Even the giving up the habit itself can cause stress that needs to be taken care of, although continuing it is also a stressor that affects negatively other areas of your life. So it's better to give it up and learn about managing stress.

For that it is helpful for you to go to a library and read books on how to manage your distress. I have a few titles for you:" The Stress Management Source Book by J. Berton Cunningham, Ph. D; Stress Owner's Manual by Ed Boenish, Ph. D., and Managing Stress by Terry Looker and Olga Gregson.

In cases where you are there is no library close by or there is no time for that, here are the basic ideas on how to manage excessive amount of tress: Terry and Olga define stress as" . a state we experience when there is mismatch between perceived demand and perceived ability to cope(If you are yourself, identify with yourself, you will feel able to cope most of the time). It is a balance on how we view demands and how we think we can cope with these demands that determines whether we feel no stress, distressed, eustress(good stress)."

It's like a reversed U curve. On the right side we have no stress or an unsignificant amount of stress, on top, we have eustress when we perform our abilities to our best, on the right side of the reversed U we have, guess what, distress or state when we are unable to perform even what we excel at. Then, when the distress is not taken care of, the person in distress becomes burnout.

- Signs of distress

irritated, overwhelmed, pressured, dissatisfied, helpless, frustrated, angry, loss of appetite, tense neck,(sleep deprivation, headache when giving up an addiction which are simply to be ignored, for they pass very quickly), etc.

- Managing distress

First of all we hope that you will not put too many irrational demands on yourself, you will be reasonable.

Second of all, it's up to you not to accept irrational demands put on you by the outer world.

Otherwise manage your state of stress by relaxation, meditation, self-hypnosis, physical exercise.

If you feel all of a sudden unhappy or mad, if you feel you might be tensed because of up-coming events, don't do physical exercise such as aerobic, running, volley ball or push ups, for a day or two, to avoid knees and or feet injuries.

L) KICKITWELL IS THE INTELLIGENCE OF ANY OTHER QUIT SMOKING DEVISE.

All you need to kick away the habit is to read the booklet utterly and apply the steps. You don't need to buy any devise. Nonetheless, if you had tried any devise before you necessarily need to use Kickitwell ,for with any quit smoking devise you will never be sure you stop for good and all. You will stop and start again any number of times, because you may not be aware of the power formation/deformation principle let alone mastering it, the smoking triggers are not controlled etc. Furthermore, some of the devises contain nicotine and nicotine produces an adverse reaction in the body's sympathetic nervous system(heart, blood vessels and sweat glands), stimulates release of fatty acid and glucose into blood.

They did this research on death crib and nicotine, and find that more infants are dying this way from cigarette smoke environment than the other way around.

And here is what a woman has said; "I used nicotine patch, but end up smoking once in a while"." I basically wanted to hit my husband with a frying pan or push him off a cliff"." I said : Don't take this personally, but I am just going to swear and yell".

So if you really want to kick the habit away, you have no other choice than to use kickitwell. Further, it's like even if you have already kicked it away spontaneously or by using some devises, you need to read this work to consolidate, to be 100% sure you quit and will not come back to it after being upset by an event somehow, if you don't want to

Use kickitwell to get rid of any unwanted habit or to form a psychological power by intensifying a desired habit. In some cases the steps in this book might need to be magnified, but every living person will benefit from reading kickitwell, be it to stop a habit, to stay away from it afterward, not to start one, or to form a psychological power.

M) How Do You Feel About the Scenery Below? It Is Disgusting, Isn'T It?

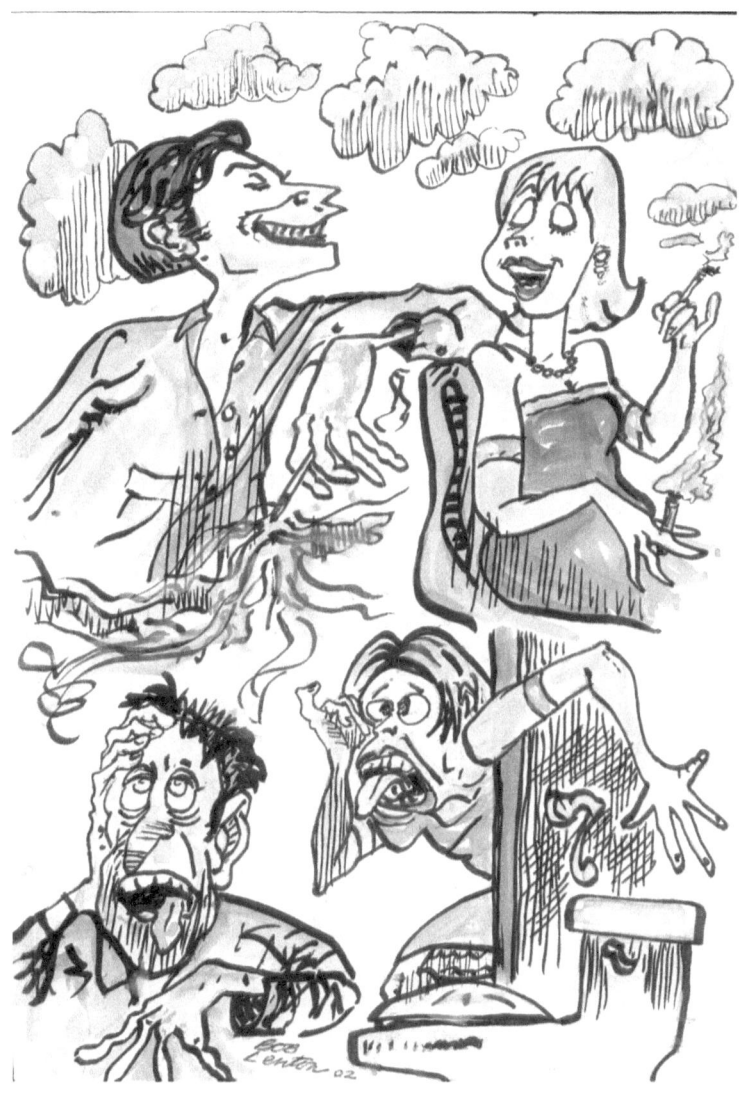

N) You Can Read My Mind and Kickitwell.

The creator of kickitwell had a class with this professor who used to tell him after course: Let's go to the smoking room. I' ll smoke; we' ll talk. After a while, I thought the professor was coming on to me sexually.

Not wanting to have an affair with her or fail the class, I tell the story to the secretary of a Dean . Instead of cooling down whatever was in her mind about me, she became overtly hysterical about it. The dean and the vice-dean of the department wrote me a letter each one asking me not to continue going to that class, to get in touch with her only through the vice-dean. In one of the last classes I had with her, she announced:" I stopped smoking". All the students applauded. Then she started talking about triggers in other context, but they are among the most important concepts in kickitwell.

The conclusion is that she had mastered the principles(or at least the principle of triggers) in kickitwell and stop smoking without reading the booklet itself, but by reading my mind. This version was not even typed yet.

After all, may be she was not in love with me, but instinctively knew I had some information she needed.

The only way for her to know about Kickitwell is by reading my mind(Not by channeling or communication between 2 dreamers, because we were not really friends). Somehow, the turmoil between her and me contributed to the mind reading. The first day in the class, I introduced myself as consecrating all my pastimes to parapsychology. I didn't say anything else; it was not a para- psychology class. But what I said, apparently, was sufficient to make her a mind reader.

That's how it becomes clear to me that you too can kick the habit away by just reading my mind (by reading kickitwell with some intensity) or by channeling, of course.

As said in the forewords, **the higher self is medicine at its** best. So raise **your consciousness level, and kick the habit away, and be healthy, and be attractive, and be rich, and be anything of value to you.**

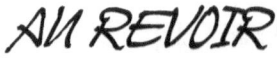

Bibliography

CUNNINGHAM J. BERTON, PH. D.

Cain Arthur. Young People and Smoking. New York: P.J.Day Company, 1964

Goldstein, Avram. M.D. Learn More Smoke Less. Lebanon N.J. 08833: Avastar Publishing Corp. 1990.

Kaplan, H. I. M.D. Comprehensive Textbook of Psychiatry. Baltimore: William Wilkins, 1981.

CREATING, ROBERT FRITZ

Petrie Sydney. How to Stop Smoking in 3 Days. New York: Warner Books Inc 1973.

Ross, Walter S How to stop Smoking Permanently with Nicotine Gum. Boston Little Brown, 1985.